DEGENERATIVE DISC DISEASE

A Beginner's 3-Step Plan to Managing DDD Through Diet and Other Natural Methods, With Sample Curated Recipes

Larry Jamesonn

mindplusfood

Copyright © 2022 Larry Jamesonn

All rights reserved

No part of this book may be reproduced, or stored in a retrieval system,
or transmitted in any form or by any means, electronic, mechanical,
photocopying, recording, or otherwise, without express written permission
of the publisher.

Printed in the United States of America

CONTENTS

Disclaimer

By reading this disclaimer, you are accepting the terms of the disclaimer in full. If you disagree with this disclaimer, please do not read the guide.

All of the content within this guide is provided for informational and educational purposes only, and should not be accepted as independent medical or other professional advice. The author is not a doctor, physician, nurse, mental health provider, or registered nutritionist/dietician. Therefore, using and reading this guide does not establish any form of a physician-patient relationship.

Always consult with a physician or another qualified health provider with any issues or questions you might have regarding any sort of medical condition. Do not ever disregard any qualified professional medical advice or delay seeking that advice because of anything you have read in this guide. The information in this guide is not intended to be any sort of medical advice and should not be used in lieu of any medical advice by a licensed and qualified medical professional.

The information in this guide has been compiled from a variety of known sources. However, the author cannot attest to or guarantee the accuracy of each source and thus should not be held liable for any errors or omissions.

You acknowledge that the publisher of this guide will not be held liable for any loss or damage of any kind incurred as a result of this guide or the reliance on any information provided within this guide. You acknowledge and agree that you assume all risk and responsibility for any action you undertake in response to the information in this guide.

Using this guide does not guarantee any particular result (e.g., weight loss or a cure). By reading this guide, you acknowledge that there are no guarantees to any specific outcome or results you can expect.

All product names, diet plans, or names used in this guide are for identification purposes only and are the property of their respective owners. The use of these names does not imply endorsement. All other trademarks cited herein are the property of their respective owners.

Where applicable, this guide is not intended to be a substitute for the original work of this diet plan and is, at most, a supplement to the original work for this diet plan and never a direct substitute. This guide is a personal expression of the facts of that diet plan.

Where applicable, persons shown in the cover images are stock photography models and the publisher has obtained the rights to use the images through license agreements with third-party stock image companies.

INTRODUCTION

Degenerative disc disease is a condition that can cause pain in the lower back and legs. It occurs when normal changes that take place in the discs of your spine cause pain. The discs are cushions between the vertebrae, and they help to absorb shock and keep the spine flexible. With age, the discs begin to degenerate or break down. This can lead to several problems, including pain, stiffness, and loss of mobility.

Degenerative disc disease is a common condition, and it is most often seen in middle-aged and older adults. Treatment typically involves analgesics or anti-inflammatory medications. In severe cases, surgery may be necessary.

While there is no cure for degenerative disc disease, there are several things that you can do to manage the pain and other symptoms. One of the most important things that you can do is to maintain a healthy lifestyle. This includes eating a healthy diet, exercising regularly, and maintaining a healthy weight.

In this quick start guide, we will give you a 3-step plan for managing degenerative disc disease through diet and other natural remedies. Specifically, we'll discuss the following in detail:

- What causes degenerative disc disease?
- What are its symptoms?

- How is it diagnosed?
- What are the treatments for degenerative disc disease?
- What are the risk factors for degenerative disc disease?
- The potential 3-step plan for managing degenerative disc disease.
- How to manage DDD through natural remedies?
- How to manage DDD through diet?
- Living with degenerative disc disease.

Without further ado, let's get started!

WHAT CAUSES DEGENERATIVE DISC DISEASE?

S everal factors can contribute to the development of degenerative disc disease. These include:

Age: The age of the patient is considered to be one of the most significant risk factors for degenerative disc disease. When you become older, the discs in your spine start to deteriorate, which is a process that can be sped up by factors such as being overweight or smoking.

Injury: A herniated disc is a kind of degenerative disc disease that can be caused by trauma to the spine. This is because the discs in your spine are designed to absorb stress, but they're still vulnerable to harm in the event of an accident.

Obesity: One of the most important contributors to the development of degenerative disc disease is obesity. This is because the additional weight places pressure on the discs in the spine, which might ultimately contribute to the degeneration of those discs.

<u>*Smoking:*</u> Additionally, smoking is a big contributor to the risk of degenerative disc degeneration. As a result, smoking reduces the amount of blood that is supplied to the discs, which might contribute to the degeneration of those discs.

WHAT ARE THE SYMPTOMS OF DDD?

D egenerative disc disease can cause several symptoms, including:

Back pain: When the discs degenerate, they lose their ability to cushion your spine and absorb shock, which can lead to pain. The pain from degenerative disc disease is typically worse with activity, such as walking or bending, and it may radiate into your legs. If you have back pain, it's important to see your doctor determine the cause.

Leg pain: The degeneration of the discs can cause several symptoms, including leg pain. The pain is typically worse with activity, and it may radiate into the back. In some cases, the pain may be so severe that it interferes with daily activities.

Stiffness: Degenerative disc disease can also cause stiffness in the back and legs. This is because the discs in the spine are designed to absorb shock, and when they degenerate, they lose this ability.

Loss of mobility: Degenerative disc disease can also lead to a loss of mobility. This is because the discs in the spine are designed to absorb shock, and when they degenerate, they lose this ability.

HOW IS DDD DIAGNOSED?

Degenerative disc disease is typically diagnosed with a physical examination and imaging tests.

Physical examination: A physical examination will be performed to assess your symptoms. This will likely include testing your range of motion and flexibility as well as checking for problems with your posture. Your doctor may also press on different areas of your spine to check for tenderness or pain. If your symptoms suggest that you may have degenerative disc disease, your doctor may order further tests, such as X-rays, MRI, or CT scans, to confirm the diagnosis.

Imaging tests: Although degenerative disc disease can be diagnosed based on a person's symptoms, imaging tests, such as x-rays, MRI, and CT scans, can be used to confirm the diagnosis. These tests can help to identify changes in the discs that are indicative of degenerative disc disease. In some cases, additional testing, such as a discogram, may be necessary to confirm the diagnosis.

Once degenerative disc disease has been diagnosed, treatment options can be discussed with a doctor.

WHAT ARE THE MEDICAL TREATMENTS FOR DEGENERATIVE DISC DISEASE?

The medical treatments for degenerative disc disease include:

Analgesics: Analgesics, such as ibuprofen and acetaminophen, can be used to relieve the pain associated with degenerative disc disease.

Anti-inflammatory medications: Anti-inflammatory medications, such as corticosteroids, can be used to reduce the inflammation associated with degenerative disc disease.

Muscle relaxants: Muscle relaxants, such as diazepam and cyclobenzaprine, can be used to relieve the muscle spasms associated with degenerative disc disease.

Narcotics: Narcotics, such as codeine and oxycodone, can be used to relieve the pain associated with degenerative disc disease.

WHAT ARE
THE SURGICAL
TREATMENTS FOR
DEGENERATIVE
DISC DISEASE?

T he surgical treatments for degenerative disc disease include:

Discectomy: Discectomy is a surgical procedure used to treat degenerative disc disease. The goal of the surgery is to remove the herniated portion of the disc and relieve the pressure on the nerves. The surgery can be performed using an open or endoscopic approach.

The open approach involves making a large incision in the back and exposing the affected area. The endoscopic approach involves making a small incision and using a special camera to visualize the affected area. Discectomy is usually performed as an outpatient procedure, meaning that the patient does not need to stay in the hospital overnight. Recovery time is typically 4-6 weeks.

Fusion: Fusion is a surgery to fuse the vertebrae. The surgeon removes the disc and replaces it with a bone graft. The fusion can be performed through an incision in the front of the spine or through a small incision in the back.

The most common type of fusion is anterior lumbar interbody fusion (ALIF). ALIF is a minimally invasive procedure that is performed through a small incision in the front of the spine. The surgeon removes the disc and replaces it with a bone graft. The fusion is then stabilized with metal hardware.

Posterior lumbar interbody fusion (PLIF) is another type of fusion that is performed through a small incision in the back. The surgeon removes the disc and replaces it with a bone graft. The fusion is then stabilized with metal hardware.

Pedicle screw fixation is a type of fixation that is used to stabilize the spine during fusion surgery. Pedicle screws are inserted into the bones of the spine and are connected to rods that run along the length of the spine. This type of fixation helps to provide stability for the spine while it heals.

Laminectomy: A laminectomy is a type of surgical procedure that is performed to remove the lamina, which is the bony plate that covers the spinal cord. This surgery is typically recommended for patients who are suffering from degenerative disc disease, as it can help to relieve pressure on the spinal cord and nerve roots.

In addition, a laminectomy may also be recommended for patients who have herniated discs or spinal stenosis. The surgical procedure itself is fairly straightforward and involves making an incision in the back so that the surgeon can access the spine. Once the surgeon has accessed the spine, they will carefully remove the lamina before closing up the incision.

In most cases, patients who undergo a laminectomy experience significant relief from their symptoms and can return to their normal activities relatively quickly.

WHAT ARE THE RISK FACTORS FOR DEVELOPING DEGENERATIVE DISC DISEASE?

The risk factors for developing degenerative disc disease include:

Age: One of the most important risk factors for degenerative disc disease is age. The discs in your spine begin to degenerate as you age, and this process is accelerated by factors such as obesity and smoking.

Injury: Spinal injuries can be extremely debilitating, and in some cases, they can also lead to degenerative disc disease. This is because the discs in the spine are designed to absorb shock, and an injury can damage them. When this happens, the discs can begin to degenerate, causing pain and stiffness.

In severe cases, the discs can collapse, putting pressure on the nerves and leading to paralysis. Degenerative disc disease is a serious condition that can significantly reduce quality of life.

Obesity: Obesity is a major risk factor for degenerative disc disease. This is because the extra weight puts pressure on the discs in the spine, and this can lead to their degeneration.

If you are obese, you should try to lose weight, as this will help to reduce your risk of degenerative disc disease. There are many ways to lose weight, and you should talk to your doctor about the best way for you. Losing even a small amount of weight can make a big difference in your risk of developing degenerative disc disease.

Smoking: Smoking is also a major risk factor for degenerative disc disease. This is because smoking decreases the blood supply to the discs, and this can lead to their degeneration.

HOW IS DEGENERATIVE DISC DISEASE PREVENTED?

Degenerative disc disease (DDD) is a condition that affects the discs in your spine. These discs are responsible for cushioning your vertebrae and helping you move around. When they become damaged, it can lead to pain, inflammation, and other problems. Fortunately, there are several things you can do to help prevent DDD from developing in the first place.

Maintaining a healthy weight: If you want to avoid degenerative disc degeneration, this is one of the most important things you can do for yourself. Maintaining a healthy weight can help to minimize your chance of developing degenerative disc disease, which is largely caused by obesity, which is a key risk factor.

Exercising: When people think of exercise, they typically envision activities like running or lifting weights. However, exercise is also crucial for maintaining the health of the spine. This is because exercise strengthens the muscles in the back and provides support for the spine. In addition, exercise helps to improve blood circulation and increase the range of motion in the spine. As a result, regular exercise can help to prevent degenerative disc disease.

Wearing supportive shoes: Wearing supportive shoes, such as low-heeled shoes, can also help to prevent degenerative disc disease. This is because high heels can put pressure on the discs in your spine and lead to their degeneration.

Avoiding smoking: Smoking damages the blood vessels in your spine, which reduces the amount of oxygen and nutrients that the discs receive. This can also contribute to disc degeneration. Avoiding smoking is one of the best things you can do to reduce your risk of degenerative disc disease. If you smoke, quitting will help to protect your spine and keep you healthy.

A 3-STEP PLAN TO MANAGING DEGENERATIVE DISC DISEASE

I t is possible to manage degenerative disc disease through diet and lifestyle changes. Here is a 3-step plan for managing degenerative disc disease:

1. Natural remedies: Some natural remedies can help to manage the symptoms of DDD. These include acupuncture, massage, exercise, diet, and yoga. Each of these treatments is effective in reducing pain and improving function.

If you are struggling with degenerative disc disease, talk to your doctor about which of these treatments may be right for you.

2. Eat a healthy diet: Eating a healthy diet is an important part of managing degenerative disc disease. There are certain foods that you should eat, and there are also certain foods that you should avoid.

3. Lifestyle changes: Making lifestyle changes is an important part of managing degenerative disc disease. These changes can include exercises to strengthen the back and lose weight. Losing weight can help to reduce the strain on the spine, and exercises that target the core muscles can help to support the spine.

In addition, avoiding smoking and maintaining good posture can also help to manage the symptoms of degenerative disc disease.

Making these changes can help to reduce the symptoms of degenerative disc disease.

NATURAL REMEDIES AND LIFESTYLE CHANGES FOR DEGENERATIVE DISC DISEASE

While there are many conventional treatments available, such as surgery and prescription medications, there are also several natural remedies that can help manage the condition. Some of these remedies include acupuncture, massage, exercise, diet, and yoga. Each of these helps relieve pain and improve function in people with degenerative disc disease.

Diet: Eating a healthy diet is one of the best things you can do for degenerative disc disease. A healthy diet includes plenty of fruits, vegetables, and whole grains. It also includes lean proteins, such as fish and chicken.

Exercise: When it comes to degenerative disc disease, exercise is an important part of the treatment plan. This is because regular exercise helps to build stronger back muscles, which provides support for the spine.

In addition, exercise helps to improve flexibility and range of motion in the spine, which can help to reduce pain. Additionally, exercise helps to increase blood flow to the discs, which helps to keep them healthy.

Finally, exercise helps to maintain a healthy weight, which puts less stress on the spine. As you can see, there are many reasons why exercise is an essential component of treating degenerative disc disease. So if you have been diagnosed with this condition, be sure to talk to your doctor about an appropriate exercise plan.

Yoga: A form of physical activity known as yoga may be beneficial in the treatment of degenerative disc disease. Because of this, the muscles in your back will become more flexible and stronger as you practice yoga. Flexibility and range of motion are two more areas that might benefit from practicing yoga. As a consequence of this, it may be able to help in the relief of pain and stiffness caused by degenerative disc disease.

Acupuncture: Acupuncture is a traditional Chinese medicine that involves inserting needles into the skin. It is believed that acupuncture can help to treat degenerative disc disease by reducing pain and inflammation.

Acupuncture is thought to work by stimulating the release of natural pain-relieving chemicals in the brain, as well as by increasing blood flow to the affected area. While acupuncture is generally considered safe, it is important to consult with a qualified practitioner to ensure that the needles are properly sterilized and inserted correctly.

Massage: While most people associate massage with relaxation, it can also be used to effectively treat a variety of conditions. One such condition is degenerative disc disease, which is characterized by the deterioration of the discs that cushion the vertebrae in your spine. This can lead to pain, inflammation, and muscle spasms.

Massage can help to reduce all of these symptoms by relaxing the muscles in your back and improving blood circulation. In addition, massage can also help to reduce inflammation by releasing adhesions between the vertebrae. As a result, massage can provide significant relief for those suffering from degenerative disc disease.

These are just a few of the natural remedies that can be used to treat degenerative disc disease. If you are interested in learning more about natural remedies for degenerative disc disease, please talk to your doctor.

MANAGING DEGENERATIVE DISC DISEASE THROUGH DIET

D egenerative disc disease is a condition that affects the spine and causes pain and stiffness in the back. While there is no cure for degenerative disc disease, there are things that you can do to manage the symptoms.

One of the most effective ways to manage degenerative disc disease is through diet. There are certain foods that you can eat to help relieve pain and stiffness, and there are also foods that you should avoid. If you have degenerative disc disease, it is important to make healthy food choices.

Foods to Eat

There are several different foods that you can eat to help relieve pain and stiffness associated with degenerative disc disease. These include:

Omega 3: Omega 3 fatty acids are a type of unsaturated fat that has many health benefits. These fats are anti-inflammatory, which means they can help to reduce pain and stiffness. They are also known for their heart-healthy properties, and they can help to lower cholesterol and blood pressure.

Omega 3 fatty acids are found in salmon, mackerel, tuna, flaxseeds, and chia seeds. All of these foods are good sources of protein, so they make a great addition to any diet. If you're looking for a way to reduce inflammation and pain, consider adding omega-3 fatty acids to your diet.

Lean protein: Muscle mass helps to support the spine, and can also help to prevent falls and other injuries. While there are many ways to encourage muscle growth, one of the most important is to include lean protein in your diet. Lean protein can be found in chicken, fish, tofu, and legumes, and provides the body with the building blocks it needs to produce new muscle tissue.

Healthy fats: One way to help prevent degenerative disc disease is to eat healthy fats. Healthy fats can be found in avocados, olive oil, nuts, and seeds. These fats help to keep the discs in your spine healthy and hydrated. They also help to reduce inflammation throughout the body. As a result, eating healthy fats can help to prevent degenerative disc disease and keep your spine healthy.

Leafy greens: Leafy greens are a good source of vitamins and minerals, and they can help to reduce inflammation. Leafy greens include spinach, kale, and Swiss chard. These greens are packed with vitamins A, C, and E, which are essential for healthy bones and joints. They also contain magnesium, potassium, and calcium. These nutrients help to reduce inflammation and improve bone health. Leafy greens can be enjoyed cooked or raw. Add them to soups, stews, salads, or smoothies for a nutrient-rich boost.

Turmeric: Turmeric is a spice that hails from South Asia and has been used in traditional medicine for centuries. The active ingredient in turmeric is curcumin, which is a powerful anti-inflammatory compound. Curcumin can help to reduce pain and stiffness, making it a popular treatment for conditions like DDD.

Turmeric can be added to food or taken as a supplement. When adding turmeric to food, it's important to note that the spice is fat-soluble, so it should be added to dishes that contain fat, such as curries or soups.

Alternatively, turmeric supplements are available in capsules or powders. It's important to consult with a healthcare provider before taking any supplements, as they can interact with other medications. When used safely, turmeric can be an effective way to reduce inflammation and pain.

By including these foods in your diet, you can help to reduce the symptoms of degenerative disc disease.

Foods to Avoid

While many foods can help to reduce pain and inflammation, some can make symptoms worse. These include:

Processed foods: Processed foods are high in unhealthy fats and chemicals, which can increase inflammation. In addition, processed foods tend to be low in nutrients that are essential for keeping bones and joints healthy. As a result, it's important to limit your intake of processed foods if you want to reduce your risk of degenerative disc disease.

Vegetable oils: It's well known that vegetable oils are high in unhealthy fats, but did you know that they can also increase inflammation? Inflammation is a major factor in degenerative disc disease, so it's important to choose your oils carefully if you're trying to protect your discs. Olive oil is the only vegetable oil that's healthy for people with degenerative disc disease.

Fried foods: When it comes to fried foods, it's not just the fat content that's cause for concern. Fried foods can increase inflammation throughout the body. Inflammation is a response by the immune system to protect against infection or injury, but when it becomes chronic, it can lead to a host of health problems.

Refined flour: Refined flour is a type of processed food that has had the bran and germ removed, leaving only the endosperm. It is then milled to create a fine, powdery texture. This type of flour is often used in baked goods, as it produces a light and airy finished product.

However, refined flour is high in unhealthy fats and chemicals. The milling process strips away many of the natural nutrients found in wheat, including fiber, vitamins, and minerals. In addition, the bleaching agents used to give refined flour its white color can damage your health.

For these reasons, it is important to limit your intake of refined flour. Choose whole-wheat alternatives whenever possible, and opt for fresh, unprocessed foods instead of processed snacks and desserts.

Sugar: Sugar can have many negative effects on the body, including inflammation and worsening symptoms of degenerative disc disease. Sugar increases inflammation by causing the body to release cytokines, which are inflammatory molecules.

In addition, sugar can alter the structure of collagen, making it more susceptible to damage. This can lead to a deterioration of the discs in the spine, which can cause pain, stiffness, and other symptoms. Therefore, it is important to limit sugar intake if you suffer from degenerative disc disease.

Avoiding these foods can help to reduce the symptoms of degenerative disc disease.

Managing degenerative disc disease through diet is an effective way to reduce pain and stiffness. There are certain foods that you should eat, and there are also certain foods that you should avoid. Making healthy food choices is an important part of managing degenerative disc disease.

SAMPLE RECIPES

<u>Vegan Caribbean Bowl</u>

Ingredients:
- 1 cup jasmine rice
- 1 cup coconut milk
- 1 cup broth
- 1 tsp. salt
- 1/4 cup unsweetened dried coconut flakes, shredded
- 4 leaves kale or collard greens, stems removed and sliced thinly
- 1/4 white cabbage, shredded
- 1/2 red bell pepper, julienned
- 1 lime, halved
- 1 tbsp. coconut oil
- 1/2 orange
- Optional: 1-2 tsp. sesame oil
- Optional, choices for garnish: avocado, carrot, cilantro lime, orange, pineapple, and/or scallion, may be combined or not

Marinade:
- 1/2 cup fresh squeezed orange juice
- 1/4 cup soy sauce
- 1 tbsp. jerk seasoning
- 1 tsp. toasted sesame oil (Asian variety)
- tempeh, cubed or sliced (may also use other protein source if desired)

Instructions:
For the marinade:
1. Mix together all the marinade ingredients.
2. Throw in the tempeh in the marinade. Let it soak for at least

half an hour.

3. In a saucepan, pour in rice, coconut milk, broth, coconut flakes, and salt.

4. Set to medium high heat and leave to boil.

5. Lower heat and allow to simmer for about 20 minutes, covered.

6. Once done, turn off the heat and leave the rice for now.

7. In a bowl, put red pepper, kale, and cabbage. Squeeze half a lime over.

8. In a pan placed over medium high heat, pour in coconut oil.

9. Add the marinated tempeh in the hot oil. Cook until all sides are cooked well.

10. Add in a teaspoon or two of sesame oil if desired. Squeeze in half an orange.

11. Remove tempeh from the pan.

12. In a serving bowl, scoop in rice, tempeh, and vegetables.

13. Upon serving, garnish according to your preference.

Baked Flounder

Ingredients:
- 1 lb. flounder, filleted
- 1/4 tsp. salt
- 1 cup halved red grapes
- 1 tbsp. extra-virgin olive oil
- 2 tbsp. parsley, chopped finely
- 1 tbsp. lemon juice
- 1 cup almonds, chopped and toasted
- freshly ground black pepper, to taste

Instructions:
1. Preheat the oven to 375°F.
2. Place fish on a sheet tray. Season with olive oil, salt, and pepper.
3. Combine the almonds, grapes, lemon juice, parsley, 1-1/2 tsp. of olive oil, 1/8 tsp of salt, and black pepper in a bowl.
4. Bake the fish for about 3 minutes.
5. Flip the fish and return to the oven.
6. Bake for another 3 minutes, or until the fish is starting to flake, while the center is still translucent. Don't overcook.
7. Serve immediately, topped with the grape mixture.

Salmon with Avocados and Brussels Sprout

Ingredients:
- 2 lbs. of salmon fillet, divided into 4 pieces
- 1 tsp. ground cumin
- 1 tsp. onion powder
- 1 tsp. paprika powder
- 1/2 tsp. garlic powder
- 1 tsp. chili powder
- Himalayan sea salt
- black pepper, freshly grounded

Avocado sauce:
- 2 chopped avocados
- 1 lime, squeezed for the juice
- 1 tbsp. extra-virgin olive oil
- 1 tbsp. fresh minced cilantro
- 1 diced small red onion
- 1 minced garlic clove
- Himalayan sea salt to taste
- black pepper, freshly grounded

Brussels sprout:
- 3 lbs. of Brussels sprout
- 1/2 cup raw honey
- 1/2 cup balsamic vinegar
- 1/2 cup melted coconut oil
- 1 cup dried cranberries
- Himalayan sea salt to taste
- black pepper, freshly grounded

Instructions:
To make the salmon and avocado sauce:
1. Combine cumin, onion, chili powder, garlic, and paprika seasoned with salt and pepper. Mix well before dry rubbing on the salmon.
2. Place the salmon in the fridge for 30 minutes.

3. Preheat the grill.
4. In a bowl, mash avocado until texture becomes smooth. Pour in all the remaining ingredients and mix thoroughly.
5. Grill salmon for 5 minutes on each side or until cooked.
6. Drizzle avocado on cooked salmon.

To make the Brussel Sprout:
1. Preheat the oven to 375 °F.
2. Mix Brussels Sprout with coconut oil. Season with salt and pepper.
3. Place vegetables on a baking sheet and roast for about 30 minutes.
4. In a separate pan, combine vinegar and honey.
5. Simmer in slow heat until it boils and thickens.
6. Drizzle them on top of the Brussels Sprouts.
7. Serve with the salmon.

Asian-Themed Macrobiotic Bowl

Ingredients:
- 2 cups cooked quinoa
- 4 carrots
- 1 package of smoked tofu
- 1 tbsp. nutritional yeast
- 2 tbsp. coconut aminos
- 4 tbsp. sunflower sprouts
- 2 tbsp. fermented vegetables
- 1 cup of shiitake mushrooms
- 1 avocado
- 2 tbsp. hemp seeds
- 2-3 cooked beets
- coconut oil cooking spray

Dressing:
- 2 tbsp. miso paste
- 1 tbsp. tahini
- 1 clove garlic, crushed
- 1 tbsp. olive oil
- 1/2 lime, juiced
- 3 tbsp. water

Instructions:
1. Roast the carrots in the oven at 400°F for 30-40 minutes.
2. Wash the vegetables, trim, and spray them with coconut oil.
3. Add them in the oven. When they are cooked, set aside till you are ready to assemble the Buddha bowl.
4. Make the dressing by combining all of the ingredients in a medium-size bowl. If the dressing appears lumpy, add more water.
5. To build the bowl, put the quinoa on the bottom and then arrange the vegetables on top.
6. Sprinkle the bowls with hemp seeds and drizzle the dressing over top.
7. Now serve and enjoy!

Chicken Salad

Ingredients:
- 1 small can premium chunk chicken breast packed in water
- 1 stalk celery, large, finely chopped
- 1/4 cup reduced-fat mayonnaise
- 4 romaine leaves or red leaf lettuce, washed and trimmed
- 8 pcs. cherry tomatoes or 1 ripe tomato, quartered
- 1 cucumber, small and sliced thinly

Instructions:
1. Drain canned chicken and transfer to a bowl.
2. Put in celery and mayonnaise.
3. Mix lightly. Don't crush the chicken.
4. In a separate shallow bowl, place the lettuce neatly.
5. Add in the chicken salad in the middle
6. Add tomatoes and cucumber slices to the plate.
7. Refrigerate before serving, cover with plastic wrap.

Baked Salmon

Ingredients:
- 2 salmon fillets
- 6 cups of fresh spinach
- 2 tsp. coconut oil
- 1/4 tsp. garlic powder
- 1/4 tsp. turmeric
- 3 large cloves of garlic
- lemon juice
- salt
- pepper

Instructions:
1. Preheat the oven to 400°F.
2. Line a baking dish with parchment paper.
3. Marinate salmon fillets in lemon juice, coconut oil, garlic powder, turmeric, salt, and pepper.
4. Let it sit for a few minutes. This may also be done the night before to help the juices and flavor get into the salmon.
5. Once the oven is ready, bake salmon for 15 minutes.
6. Cook some of the garlic in a pan with coconut oil.
7. Add spinach and cook until ready. Season with salt and pepper to taste.
8. Take salmon out of the oven and put spinach beside it.
9. Serve and enjoy.

Asian Zucchini Salad

Ingredients:
- 1 medium zucchini, sliced thinly into spirals
- 1/3 cup rice vinegar
- 3/4 cup avocado oil
- 1 cup sunflower seeds, shells removed
- 1 lb. cabbage, shredded
- 1 tsp. stevia drops
- 1 cup almonds, sliced

Instructions:
1. Cut the zucchini spirals into smaller parts. Set aside.
2. Put almonds, sunflower seeds, and cabbage in a large bowl. Combine the ingredients well.
4. Add zucchini to the mixture.
5. In a small bowl, mix vinegar, stevia, and oil using a whisk or fork.
6. Pour vinegar mixture all over the zucchini mixture. Toss well. Make sure everything is covered with the dressing.
7. Refrigerate for 2 hours before serving.

Low FODMAP Burger

Ingredients:
- 1-1/4 lbs. ground pork
- 1/4 tsp. allspice
- 1/2 tsp. salt
- 1/2 tsp. white pepper
- 1/2 tsp. ground nutmeg
- 1/2 tsp. caraway seeds
- 1/2 tsp. ground ginger

Instructions:
1. Preheat the grill then prepare the patty.
2. Using a small mixing bowl, stir together the salt, pepper, allspice, nutmeg, and ginger until fully combined.
3. Place the ground in a large mixing bowl and add the spice mixture.
4. Mix thoroughly until spices are evenly distributed to the pork.
5. Make round, flat burger patties using the palm of your hands.
6. Grill the patties and serve with gluten-free buns and mustard sauce.

Stir-Fried Cabbage and Apples

Ingredients:
- 1 shallot, thinly sliced
- 1/2 apple, cut into cubes
- 1/4 savoy cabbage, sliced thinly into strips
- 3–4 radishes, sliced thinly
- 1/2–1 tsp. coconut oil
- salt, to taste

Instructions:
1. Pour some coconut oil into a wok.
2. Add shallot and cook until translucent.
3. Add the cabbage, radish, and apples to the wok.
4. Stir-fry for about 5 minutes. Don't overcook.
5. Add salt to taste.
6. Serve while warm.

Asparagus and Greens Salad with Tahini and Poppy Seed Dressing

Ingredients:
- 10 to 12 asparagus stalks, washed well and sliced into ribbons
- 5 radishes, washed well, and sliced thinly
- 2 to 3 rainbow carrots, peeled and sliced thinly
- 1 handful wild spinach
- 1 small handful of microgreens, washed well
- 1 small handful of sunflower greens, washed well
- optional: few pieces of chive blossoms

For the dressing:
- 2 tbsp. tahini
- 1 tbsp. poppy seeds
- 1 tbsp. extra-virgin olive oil
- salt
- pepper

Instructions:
1. For the dressing, whisk ingredients together in a small bowl.
2. In a separate bowl, toss salad ingredients in the mixture.
3. Drizzle dressing on salad upon serving.

Stir-Fried Cabbage and Apples

Ingredients:
- 1 shallot, thinly sliced
- 1/2 apple, cut into cubes
- 1/4 savoy cabbage, sliced thinly into strips
- 3–4 radishes, sliced thinly
- 1/2–1 tsp. coconut oil
- salt, to taste

Instructions:
1. Pour some coconut oil into a wok.
2. Add shallot and cook until translucent.
3. Add the cabbage, radish, and apples to the wok.
4. Stir-fry for about 5 minutes. Don't overcook.
5. Add salt to taste.
6. Serve while warm.

Roasted Chicken Thighs

Ingredients:
- 12 garlic cloves, unpeeled
- 1 tbsp. avocado oil
- 1 pinch Himalayan pink salt
- 4 chicken thighs with skin
- 1 tsp. Primal Palate super gyro seasoning

Instructions:
1. Pour avocado oil over a medium-sized oven-safe pot.
2. Add the garlic cloves. Sauté over medium heat for 2 to 3 minutes or until the skins begin to brown.
3. Place the chicken in a large skillet over medium-high heat. Sear for about 2 to 3 minutes for each side, starting with the skin side.
4. Combine the chicken with the garlic. Season generously with salt and Primal Palate Super Gyro seasoning.
5. Place the chicken in an oven preheated to 350°F.
6. Bake for one hour while covered.
7. Serve and enjoy.

Arugula and Mushroom Salad

Ingredients:
- 5 oz. arugula washed
- 1 lb. fresh mushrooms
- 1/4 tsp. shoyu
- 1/2 red onion
- 1 tbsp. olive oil
- 1 tbsp. mirin

For tofu cheese:
- 1/8 cup umeboshi vinegar
- 1/2 firm tofu

Instructions:
1. In a bowl, add the rinsed tofu. Crumble and pour in vinegar.
2. In a separate bowl add shoyu, red onions, salt, olive oil, and mirin. 3. Mix to combine.
4. Add in the arugula and toss to combine with the dressing.
5. Serve and enjoy.

Cauliflower and Mushroom Bake

Ingredients:
- 3 cups cauliflower florets
- 1 cup fresh mushroom, chopped
- 1/2 cup red onion, chopped
- 1/3 cup green onion, chopped
- 2 garlic cloves, finely chopped
- 2 tsp. apple cider vinegar
- 2 tsp. lemon juice
- 1/2 tsp. salt
- 1/4 tsp. pepper
- 1 tbsp. olive oil

Instructions:
1. Preheat the oven to 350°F. Lightly grease a baking pan.
2. Combine red onion, cauliflower, olive oil, garlic, mushroom, apple cider vinegar, lemon juice, salt, and pepper in a bowl. Mix well.
3. Pour the mixture into the greased baking pan.
4. Place inside the oven and bake for 45 minutes. Stir.
5. When vegetables are golden brown and tender, remove from the oven.
6. Garnish with green onions. Serve and enjoy.

Living with Degenerative Disc Disease

If you have degenerative disc disease, it is important to take care of yourself. There are things that you can do to manage the symptoms and make your life easier.

Managing Pain: There are several ways that you can manage pain. Pain medication can be used to relieve pain, but it is important to use pain medication as directed by your doctor. You can also use ice or heat to relieve pain, and you can try stretching exercises.

Exercise: Exercise is an important part of managing degenerative disc disease. Exercise helps to strengthen the muscles that support the spine. It also helps to increase flexibility and range of motion. When you exercise, it is important to start slowly and to increase the intensity gradually.

Managing Stress: Stress can make the symptoms of degenerative disc disease worse. There are several ways that you can manage stress. You can try relaxation techniques, such as yoga or meditation. You can also try to get regular exercise, and you can spend time with friends and family.

Making Lifestyle Changes: There are several lifestyle changes that you can make to manage degenerative disc disease. You can quit smoking, and you can limit your alcohol intake. You can also try to lose weight, and you can make sure that you are getting enough sleep.

Degenerative disc disease can be a painful condition. There are things that you can do to manage the pain and make your life easier. By following these tips, you can help to improve your quality of life.

Conclusion

Degenerative disc disease can be a painful condition, but there are things that you can do to manage the pain and make your life easier. Eating a healthy diet, getting regular exercise, and managing stress are all important parts of managing degenerative disc disease.

Making lifestyle changes, such as quitting smoking and losing weight, can also help to improve your quality of life. If you're dealing with degenerative disc disease, talk to your doctor about ways to manage your pain and improve your quality of life.

This article is for informational purposes only and is not intended to be a substitute for medical advice, diagnosis, or treatment. If you have any concerns or questions about your health, you should always consult with a healthcare professional.

References

https://spinehealth.org/nutrition-for-degenerative-disc-disease/
https://my.clevelandclinic.org/health/diseases/16912-degenerative-disk-disease
https://www.cedars-sinai.org/health-library/diseases-and-conditions/d/degenerative-disc-disease.html#:~:text=Degenerative%20disc%20disease%20isn't,daily%20activities%2C%20sports%20and%20injuries.
https://www.csiortho.com/blog/2018/september/7-foods-you-need-to-be-eating-for-spinal-health/
https://www.medicalnewstoday.com/articles/266630#symptoms
https://spinenation.com/conditions/degenerative-disc-disease/foods-to-avoid-that-increase-inflammation-back-pain
https://www.versusarthritis.org/about-arthritis/complementary-and-alternative-treatments/types-of-complementary-treatments/vitamins-a-c-and-e/

.

Made in the USA
Monee, IL
09 June 2023

35538219R00030